Comments about

SAVE YOUR LIFE

"This book fulfills a real need."

–Jeff Flier, M.D.
Dean, Harvard Medical School

"This book is filled with important information that everyone should have at their fingertips."

–Suzanne Andrews of PBS TV's
Functional Fitness Starring Suzanne Andrews

"About as comprehensive a guide as one could imagine. It should be required reading and kept handy at every school, summer camp, health club, senior center, hotel, and any other place of public accommodation."

–Charles H. Baron, LL.B., Ph.D.
Professor of Law Emeritus
Boston College Law School

"This should be required reading for young and old alike."

–Ruth Harriet Jacobs, Ph.D., former AARP's
National Task Force on Aging and Mental Health program

"I would recommend that it be reading for all high school seniors or college freshman. It is well written and has potential for great practical value."

–George E. Altman, M.D.

"This book fulfills a need to have important health solutions close at hand. I recommend it for people of all ages."

–Lois Landau Berman, J.D., LL.M

"Having read the book, I feel better prepared for anything that might happen."

–Simon Posniakoff, retired navigator, El Al Airlines

"This is an important book that tells you what to do in a medical emergency. Everyone should have it."

–Mrs. Naomi Spector, retired business owner

"This book is packed with an incredible amount of easy-to-understand and useful information. It is a great resource that no home should be without."

–Bryan Davis, professional editor

SAVE YOUR LIFE...

What to Do In a Medical Emergency

Shelly Glazier, M.Ed., LMFT
Mache Seibel, M.D.

Wolff Publishing
Newton, MA

Every effort has been made to ensure that the information in this book is complete and accurate. This book is intended only as an informative guide for those wishing to know more about health issues. In no way is this book intended to replace, countermand, or conflict with the advice given to you by your own physician.

The ultimate decision concerning care should be made between you and your doctor. We strongly recommend you follow his or her advice.

Information in this book is general and is offered with no guarantees on the part of the authors or Save Your Life Book, LLC. The authors and publisher disclaim all liability in connection with the use of this book.

The names and identifying details of people associated with events described in this book have been changed. Any similarity to actual persons is coincidental.

ISBN 978-0-615-43737-8

Library of Congress Control Number: 1-550811991
Cover and illustrations by
Darren Wheeling-Black Egg Syndicate

Dedicated with love to Bill, a wonderful husband, father, grandfather, and father-in-law; a man of compassion, strength, and sensitivity whose devotion to medicine and caring for children and their families was unending.

Shelly

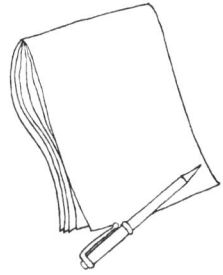

This Medical Guide Belongs To:

Name: _____

Date of Birth: _____

In A Medical Emergency Please
Give This Guide To:

Name: _____

Relationship: _____

Home Phone: _____

Cell Phone: _____

Acknowledgements

I would like to thank the many people who attended my classes, *What is a Medical Emergency* at Brandeis University's BOLLI Program; they were my inspiration for writing this book. Their personal stories on how the course helped them, made me realize the need for an easy to read and understand book.

It is with great appreciation that I want to thank my son-in-law, Mache Seibel, M.D., for his collaboration and help in the writing of this book. His patience, as we wrote, edited and re-edited was above and beyond the call of duty.

My wonderful daughter, Sharon Seibel, M.D., deserves my deepest thanks for her constructive help and feedback. I also want to thank Kenneth Glazier, M.D., his wife, Susan, Arnold Glazier, M.D. his wife Maryann, and their daughter, Roxy, all of whom offered thoughtful comments and advice.

I would like to thank my dear friends, Dr. Ruth Harriet Jacobs, Simon Posniakoff, and Alan Glou who graciously read drafts and offered many helpful comments. I would also like to thank Brian Davis and Dr. Robert Barasch who helped edit the original text.

A special thanks to Allen Glazier for his meticulous and outstanding editorial and formatting assistance. –SG

~

To Sharon, my wife, best friend, advisor and biggest fan who made completing this book possible. Thank you. –MS

Table of Contents

Chapter 1

What's a Medical Emergency?

It is three a.m. and you or your loved one awakes with one or more of the following symptoms:

- A cold sweat

- A sense of doom or a feeling that something bad is going to happen

- Mild chest pain

- Extreme restlessness

- Extreme fatigue

- Faintness

- A feeling of being sick in the stomach, vomiting

- Nausea, lightheadedness

- Pain in one or both arms

- Pain in the neck, jaw, or stomach

- Unexplained back pain

- Upper body discomfort

What Do You Think Is The Problem?

Mark the box that you think has the correct answer.

[ ]　The flu

[ ]　Indigestion (upset stomach)

[ ]　A heart attack

The answer is...

It could be all of the above! These multiple symptoms *could* indicate something as minor as an upset stomach, but also could be something as serious as a heart attack.

If you think you *might* be having a medical emergency like a heart attack, call 9-1-1.

Here are four important questions and their answers that you should know if you think there could be a medical emergency:

Should you…

1. Call your doctor?

   No! Waiting for the doctor to call back wastes valuable time.

2. Rest to see if you feel better?

   No! Waiting to see if the symptoms pass also wastes time that could save a life. The sooner you get medical care, the more likely you are to live.

3. Drive yourself to the hospital?

   No! If you drive yourself to the hospital, you might pass out or stop breathing on the way.

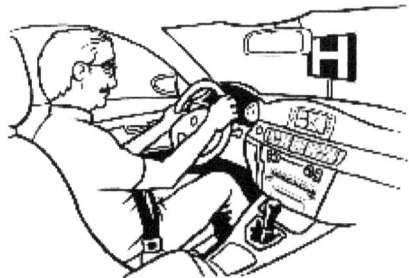

4. Call your family or friend for a ride to the hospital?

    No! Do not ask family or friends to drive you to the hospital (unless emergency services are unavailable). If you lose consciousness, your driver likely won't be able to help you.

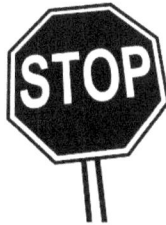

In all of these cases, you should call 9-1-1 immediately.

When you call 9-1-1, the responding Emergency Medical Technicians (EMTs) will monitor you. If you stop breathing or your heart stops beating, they will give you emergency treatment on the way to the hospital. They also will notify the emergency room staff of your condition, so when you arrive they will know you need immediate treatment.

Calling 9-1-1 is the safest and fastest way to get medical care. Remember, car accidents are more likely to happen when family or friends are trying to rush you to the hospital.

People Often Ask…

I've had many of the symptoms you mentioned at one time or another, how will I know when to call 9-1-1?

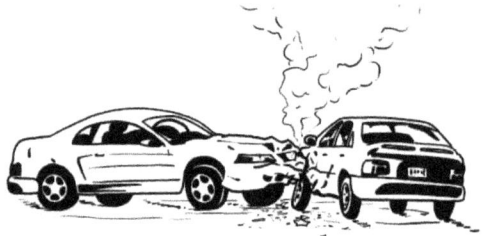

The Answer Is…

Everyone knows how his or her own body normally feels. When your body starts to feel very unusual or strange, don't try to diagnose the symptoms on your own.

Call 9-1-1 immediately!

For example, if you experience a sudden onset of extreme fatigue or any other symptoms that you've never felt before, don't ignore it. If you think it could be life threatening, or you're not sure, don't guess… Call 9-1-1.

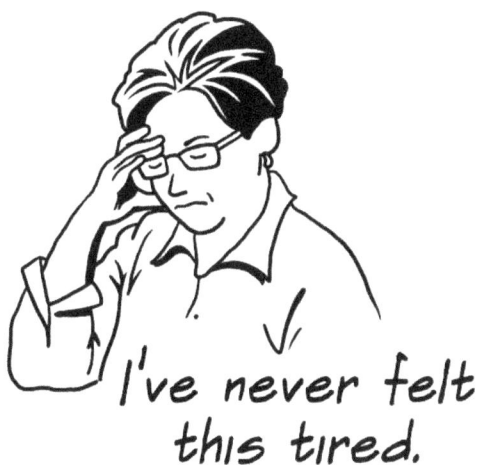

I've never felt this tired.

You Call 9-1-1...Then What?

While it is important to know **when** to call 9-1-1 for help, the following are ten important things to keep in mind **after** you have called.

1. Unlock the front door so EMTs can quickly get into your house without breaking down your door.

2. Turn on inside and outside lights at night to help the EMTs and ambulance find your house faster.

3. Restrain dogs or other pets that might prevent emergency providers from reaching the patient quickly

4. Remove cars and furniture that are blocking the way to make room for a stretcher.

5. Have someone meet the emergency crews and take them directly to the patient.

6. Have your cell phone available, with your *In Case of Emergency* (ICE) numbers. (See page 16 for more information on ICE).

7. Take your *Medication, Allergy and Doctor* (MAD) list (see page 17 for more information on MAD).

8. Take your insurance cards.

9. If possible, call your family, a friend, or neighbor and tell them which hospital you're being taken to.

10. Call your doctor, if possible.

What if you have a medical emergency and are by yourself in a crowded area and unable to call 9-1-1? Studies show the best thing to do is point to one person, tell them you are having a medical emergency, and ask them to call 9-1-1 for you. By doing this, you make it clear that you are in need of help, and are both asking and depending on that person to help you. That is the most effective way of obtaining assistance from a stranger in a crowded situation.[1]

Submit *your* medical emergency story or experience, and find recommended website links at: www.saveyourlifebook.com

---

[1] Source: *Influence: The Psychology of Persuasion,* by Robert B. Cialdini. P 138

Eight Reasons People Do Not Call 9-1-1 During a Medical Emergency:

1. Someone tells them not to call

2. They don't want to bother anyone

3. They think their condition is not serious, and feel they will look foolish calling 9-1-1

4. They think if they just wait they will feel better

5. They don't want to wait in the emergency room

6. They think they should talk to their doctor before calling 9-1-1

7. They think they cannot afford the medical expense of going to the hospital

8. They're in the middle of a good TV program

It doesn't matter if someone doesn't want you to call for help. If you think it's an emergency, don't take "No" for an answer.

Call 9-1-1.

A Personal Lesson

I learned to say, "Yes, dear," and dial 9-1-1 anyway when my late husband Bill, a physician, had a medical emergency.

One evening Bill came home extremely tired; he barely ate dinner. This was very unusual for him. He wanted to rest and headed for his easy chair. He never made it. Without warning, he collapsed.

I told him, "I'm calling 9-1-1" "No, No," he said, "I just need to rest a bit." I was extremely worried, so I said, "I'm calling Ken," our son, also a physician, who lived next door. "Don't bother Ken," Bill said, "I'm fine." When I looked at him, I felt he wasn't fine at all, and decided to call our son.

Ken asked if I had called 9-1-1. I told him I hadn't because Dad didn't want me to. He immediately called 9-1-1 and came right over.

Later, I learned Bill could have died without emergency treatment. My experience taught me that even doctors could make the wrong decision when personally experiencing a medical emergency. It's known as being in denial.

Ken told me this could happen again and if Dad didn't want me to call 9-1-1 to just say, "Yes, dear," and dial 9-1-1. –SG

If you feel there could be a serious medical problem and you are alone, don't wait. Follow your instincts and **call 9-1-1.**

Remember; **never** waste time in an emergency. Always call **9-1-1** first and then, if possible, unlock the door and turn on the lights. You can then call your family, friends, and doctor.

You will not look foolish! Even if you think you will, it's better to call 9-1-1 than later wish you had done so. You could be saving your life or someone else's.

If your loved one doesn't want you to call for help, don't argue with them! Just say, "Yes, dear," or "OK," and dial 9-1-1 anyway. They'll thank you later.

Chapter 2

Help Others Help You

There are two valuable pieces of information EMTs need when treating a patient, especially when the patient cannot communicate with them:

1. Whom to contact in an emergency

2. The patient's medical information

You can help those who are trying to help you by having your *In Case of Emergency* (**ICE**) contacts listed in your cell phone and by having your medical history available in a *Medication, Allergy and Doctor* (**MAD**) list.

Keep a copy of your MAD list in your purse or wallet and on your refrigerator. First responders know to look there for information.

ICE Telephone Numbers

After you call 9-1-1 it is extremely helpful to have your cell phone available with your ICE numbers.

In

Case of

Emergency

These ICE numbers could be the most important phone numbers you have in your cell phone's contact list because they are the people you want called in an emergency. EMTs know to look for and call ICE numbers in a medical crisis. Setting up your ICE numbers in your phone is easy to do and could prove invaluable in an emergency.

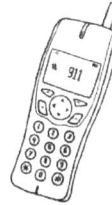

Setting Up Your ICE Contacts

The first two contact numbers in your cell phone's contact list should be for the people you want called in an emergency (make sure those people know your medical history). Enter "ICE" and then your emergency contact names.

For Example:

- **ICE...Dan 617-000-0000**

- **ICE...Sue 781-000-0000**

Emergency medical personnel will know to call them if you are unable to communicate. In addition to setting up your ICE numbers so they are the first two numbers in your contact list, you can set them up in the order in which you would like them called, such as "ICE 1" and "ICE 2."

For Example:

- **ICE 1...Tom 781-000-0000**

- **ICE 2...Ann 617-000-0000**

Your MAD List

Another very valuable piece of information EMTs look for is a list of your:

MEDICATIONS
ALLERGIES
DOCTORS

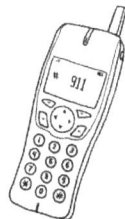

Your **MAD** list is extremely important because it gives the emergency team vital medical information they will need to properly care for you.

It's also helpful to add a note in your MAD list if you have any special medical devices, such as a pacemaker.

Please see pages 143 to149 for MAD list forms that you can fill out and personalize.

Having your ICE contacts set up in your cell phone and your MAD list complete are simple things you can do to help medical emergency personnel help you.

Chapter 3

Heart Attacks

Two of the most serious medical emergencies that people often don't recognize are heart attacks and strokes. The signs for each can be subtle or severe so it's important to recognize when medical attention is needed.

A heart attack is a mechanical problem caused by blockage of the heart's blood vessels. There isn't enough blood flow to the heart and cardiac muscle dies. Many people think if someone is having a heart attack they will have terrible chest pain and collapse. However, there are many other symptoms that may signal a heart attack. Women often have very subtle signs of a heart attack that can easily be missed. Often they don't even seek medical care.

Each year approximately 1.2 million Americans suffer heart attacks. That's about one person every 30 seconds. It's crucial to recognize signs of a heart attack and call 9-1-1 immediately.[2]

---

[2] www.cdc.gov/dhdsp/data_statistics/fact_sheets/docs/fs_state_heartattack.pdf

Julia's Story

Julia's experience is an example of how a subtle sign can signal a serious medical problem. Julia was 59 years old, slim, exercised regularly, ate well, and had never been really sick.

One evening while getting ready for bed, she told her husband, Colin, that she felt extremely restless. She didn't know why she felt that way, but decided to sleep on the couch so she wouldn't bother him.

At 4:30 a.m., Colin awoke when he heard a loud groan. He found Julia unconscious. Colin immediately called 9-1-1, and was told how to perform CPR, which he did, until the emergency team arrived.

Julia had a blood clot to her heart and was in a coma for several days. Because Colin called 9-1-1 immediately and performed CPR as directed, Julia is alive and in good health today. –SG

You may wonder how Julia could have known that her feeling of extreme restlessness was a sign of a heart problem. The key is the word **extreme**; that's what made it a major warning sign. Feeling that way was not normal for Julia.

Symptoms of a Heart Attack

The most common symptoms of a heart attack include:

- A cold sweat

- A sick feeling in the stomach, vomiting

- Discomfort in the upper body

- Extreme fatigue

- Extreme restlessness, a sense of doom, or feeling something bad is about to happen

- Mild chest pain or unexplained back pain

- Nausea, dizziness, or fainting

- Pain in one or both arms

- Pain in the neck, jaw, or stomach

What to Do During a Heart Attack

Is taking an aspirin helpful if you are having a heart attack? The most important thing to do if you think you are having a heart attack is **call 9-1-1** at once.[3]

After that, chew one adult 325 mg aspirin, which can lower your chance of dying from a heart attack.

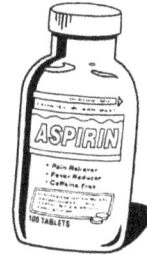

Exception: Five Reasons Not Take Aspirin

1. You are allergic to aspirin.

2. Your doctor warned you not to take aspirin because of other medications you are taking.

3. Aspirin makes other conditions you have worse.

4. You have a bleeding problem or think you're bleeding internally.

5. You think you are having a stroke.

---

[3] www.mayoclinic.com/health/first-aid-heart-attack/FA00050

Chapter 4

Sudden Cardiac Arrest

Sudden cardiac arrest (SCA) is different from a heart attack. It is an electrical problem. The heart's electrical system causes it to either pump irregularly (arrhythmia) or suddenly stop pumping altogether. This causes blood to stop flowing to the brain and other vital organs. The person becomes unconsciousness, stops breathing, and has no signs of life. If not treated, death occurs within minutes.[4] Unlike a heart attack, which generally happens to older people, sudden cardiac arrest can happen at any age, even to professional athletes.

---

[4] <http://www.nhlbi.nih.gov/health/dci/Diseases/scda/scda_whatis.html>

Automated External Defibrillator (AED)

Over 325,000 Americans die of sudden cardiac arrest every year.[5] There is now a device called an Automated External Defibrillator (AED) that can help save a victim of cardiac arrest.

An AED is a small, computerized device that analyzes heart rhythm to detect cardiac arrest. It helps re-establish a normal heart rhythm by delivering a high-energy electrical shock, if needed, through paddles or electrodes that have been applied to the victim's chest.

A voice prompt, lights and text messages automatically tells the rescuer exactly what to do. When AEDs are used along with CPR, they can increase survival rates by 50 percent.[6] AEDs are safe and effective.

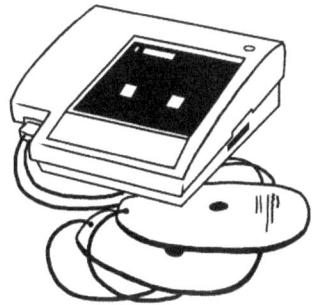

It will not shock someone who does not need to be shocked.

---

[5] http://www.heartrhythmfoundation.org/facts/scd.asp

[6] http://www.americanheart.org/presenter.jhtml?identifier=4483

How to Deal With Cardiac Arrest

1. Immediately call **9-1-1.**

2. Perform hands only CPR (see pages 132-133).

3. If you're in a public setting, have someone immediately look for an (AED), which is marked with this sign.

4. Use the AED as instructed by the device until help arrives.

Don't worry. It's easy to do. In a study, untrained sixth-grade students were able to perform defibrillation correctly with an AED in about 90 seconds.[7] AED's are now commonly found at shopping malls, restaurants, schools, health clubs, businesses, and on trains and airplanes.

---

[7] Gundry JW, Comess KA, DeRook FA et al. Comparison of Naive Sixth-Grade Children With Trained Professionals in the Use of an Automated External Defibrillator. Circulation. 1999; 100:1703-1707.

Timing Is Everything

The day started normally for Jason, a seemingly healthy man of 48. However, it turned out to be anything but normal. He had just arrived at the local high school for a meeting with his son's teacher when he suddenly collapsed and stopped breathing.

Call it fate, a miracle, or whatever else you like, but a new AED device had been delivered to the school that morning, and the staff had just finished watching a demonstration of how it worked. When Jason collapsed, one of the teachers immediately called 9-1-1. Another teacher grabbed the AED and used it to bring Jason back to life.

What could have been a tragedy ended happily for everyone involved. –SG

Chapter 5

Striking Back at Stroke

A stroke is a very real emergency. Every 40 seconds someone in the United States has a stroke and approximately every three minutes someone dies from a stroke.[8] The brain is the body's computer and it needs a good blood supply and enough oxygen to function properly. When the brain doesn't get enough oxygen, brain cells die quickly.

---

[8] "CDC - DHDSP - Stroke Facts." Centers for Disease Control and Prevention. Web. 15 Dec. 2010. <http://www.cdc.gov/stroke/facts.htm>.

Common Symptoms of Stroke

The National Stroke Association's "ACT FAST©" list can help you identify the symptoms of a stroke:

FACE   Ask the person to smile. Does one side of the face droop?

ARMS   Ask the person to raise both arms. Does one arm drift downward?

SPEECH   Ask the person to repeat a simple sentence. Ask them to repeat a phrase. Are the words slurred or strange?

TIME   If the person shows any of these symptoms, time is important because brain cells die every second.

Call 9-1-1 or, if not available, go to a hospital immediately at *any* sign of a stroke.

Other Symptoms of Stroke

In addition to the previously mentioned symptoms of a stroke, other signs can include sudden:[9]

- Confusion

- Difficulty seeing with one or both eyes

- Flopping of tongue to one side or not able to stick tongue out

- Loss of balance or coordination

- Lost, blurry or double vision

- Numbness or weakness of the face, arms or legs

- Problems walking or dizziness

- Severe headache with or without known cause

- Trouble speaking or understanding others

Always call 9-1-1 when there are signs of a stroke, even if they seem to go away. People can suffer a mini-stroke,

---

[9] http://www.stroke.org/site/PageServer?pagename=symp

which can go away after a few minutes, but one in five times it will be followed by a major stoke in the next three months. Don't wait until it's too late.

Always check the time when the first warning sign or symptom of a stroke was noticed. It is vital information the medical team will need to know, since certain medications can only be given within a certain period of time, usually three hours, after the first stroke symptoms occur.[10]

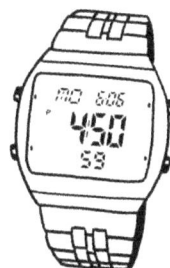

Although strokes are often associated with older people, strokes can and do occur at *any* age; consider that nearly 25% of strokes occur in people under the age of 65. Young people, mainly those who have heart problems, diabetes, and/or high blood pressure, are at risk for stroke, especially if they are African-American. Stroke is *always* an emergency.[11]

---

[10] "CDC - DHDSP - Stroke Facts." Centers for Disease Control and Prevention. Web. 15 Dec. 2010. <http://www.cdc.gov/stroke/facts.htm>.

[11] NCHS publication National Vital Statistics Report: Deaths: Preliminary Data for 2003 (NVSR, 2005; 53:15)

When it comes to strokes, "sudden" is important because stroke symptoms happen very suddenly. Many people have more than one symptom at the same time.

Do not wait to see if the symptoms go away. Even if they do, the person may be having a stroke. **Call 9-1-1** immediately.[12]

Submit *your* medical emergency story or experience, and find recommended website links at: www.saveyourlifebook.com

[12] http://www.ninds.nih.gov/disorders/stroke/knowstroke.htm

Other Medical Emergencies

There are many other common medical emergencies in addition to heart attacks and stroke, including:

- Allergic reactions
- Asthma
- Bleeding
- Burns
- Choking
- Diabetes
- Falls and slips
- Head injuries
- Meningitis
- Poisoning
- Seizures
- Shortness of breath

Let's review these emergencies next. As with any medical-related issues, knowing what to look for will help you decide if and when you should call 9-1-1 for help.

Chapter 6

Allergic Reactions

At one time or another, many people have an allergic reaction to something they have eaten or come in contact with. It is generally little more than a nuisance and their doctor can tell them what medication they should use. However, in a severe allergic reaction, difficulty breathing and other serious symptoms can happen quickly. These symptoms are called anaphylaxis, which is a critical medical emergency that, if untreated, can lead to death.

If you think someone is having a severe allergic reaction or anaphylaxis and cannot wake him or her up call 9-1-1 immediately. Also, call if they are awake but seem confused.

Signs of a Serious Allergic Reaction[13]

- Loss of consciousness

- Trouble breathing or wheezing

- Hives (raised welts), itching

- Fear or feeling of apprehension or anxiety

- Dizziness

- Swelling in the face, eyelids, lips, tongue, throat, hands, and feet

- Chest discomfort or tightness

- Weakness

- Palpitations

- Flushing or redness of the face

- Difficulty swallowing

- Cramps, abdominal pain, diarrhea

---

[13] http://www.nlm.nih.gov/medlineplus/ency/article/000005.htm

The following is a story of what happened to a friend of mine when she was simply stung by a bee.

Allergic Reactions to a Bee Sting

Many years ago, my friend Lila called to ask for advice because she had just been stung by a bee and was covered in welts. She didn't know what to do.

I told her to get immediate medical care because bee stings could cause a fatal reaction. She said I was overacting; it was just a bee sting.

About a half hour later when I called to check on her, her neighbor, Emily, answered the phone. Emily had stopped by for a cup of coffee. When no one answered and she heard the children crying inside, she knew something was wrong.

She immediately called the police (this was before cell phones and 9-1-1). When they arrived Lila was lying on the floor unconscious. Emily's quick thinking and the fast actions of the police saved Lila's life. –SG

Did you know that many people can be seriously affected by airborne allergens such as animal hair, latex, chemical vapors and certain foods like peanuts? Just breathing these particles in the air can cause a serious reaction. If someone is having a serious reaction to an airborne allergen, immediately remove them from area. If it's available, inject them with an Epi-Pen©, a syringe filled with epinephrine (adrenaline), to help treat the allergic reaction. Then call 9-1-1.

Six Common Things That Can Cause Allergic Reactions

1. Foods like shellfish, fish, nuts

2. Latex (natural rubber)

3. Prescription and over-the-counter medications

4. Transfusion of blood or blood products

5. Venom from stinging insects like yellow jackets, bees, wasps, or fire ants

6. X-ray dyes used during procedures or tests

People with asthma, eczema, or hay fever are slightly more likely to have severe allergic reactions than others.

Peanut Allergy

When my son's friend Tom visited for the first time, Tom's mother brought an Epi-Pen©, which is a syringe filled with epinephrine (adrenaline). She told me the boy had many allergies, and was very allergic to peanuts. She wanted me to have the Epi-Pen© immediately available should he have a severe allergic reaction to anything in the house.

She warned me that since he was highly allergic to peanuts, if there was even peanut dust in the air, he could have a serious reaction and be unable to breathe. Tom didn't go anywhere without his Epi-Pen. Injecting him with the Epi-Pen©, she said, could save his life. –MS

This may seem like a lot of fuss over a possible allergic reaction, but for people like Tom, it can be a matter of life or death. If you have a food allergy, and are eating out, *always* ask your server if what you are ordering contains the food or spices you are allergic to.

Chapter 7

Asthma

Asthma makes it difficult, or at times, impossible for people to breathe properly. Their lungs wheeze, and they may need to use an inhaler to help them breathe normally, especially before they exercise, or if they have a cold.

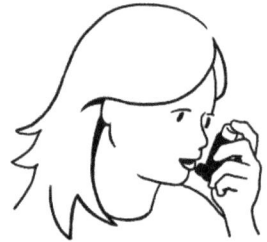

Asthma usually can be controlled with rest and prescription medications. To help prevent a severe asthma attack, symptoms should be treated as soon as they are noticed.

When asthma symptoms become worse than usual, breathing can become so difficult that the person can die from lack of oxygen. Asthma kills 4,000 people a year or 11 people every day.[14]

---

[14] New Asthma Estimates: Tracking Prevalence, Health Care and Mortality," NCHS, CDC, 2001

Don't let that happen to you or your loved one. Don't wait until it's too late. **Call 9-1-1** if there are symptoms of acute asthma or if the asthma attack doesn't respond to rest and medication as quickly as usual.

Symptoms of Acute Asthma

- Blue lips or fingernails

- Chest pain or pressure

- Coughing with asthma that won't stop

- Difficulty talking

- Feelings of anxiety or panic

- Low peak flow readings when using a peak flow meter

- Pale, sweaty face

- Severe wheezing when breathing in or out

- Symptoms that worsen, even though medications are being used

- Tightened neck and chest muscles, called retractions

- Very rapid breathing

At the hospital, an asthma patient will be closely monitored and given oxygen and proper medication. Calling 9-1-1 can save a life.

Symptoms of Common Asthma

- **Chest tightness:** it feels like someone is squeezing or sitting on your chest

- **Coughing:** it is often worse at night or early morning, making it difficult to sleep

- **Shortness of breath:** feeling unable to catch a breath or feeling out of breath

- **Wheezing:** a whistling or squeaky sound when breathing

Remember: Always call a doctor or go to the emergency room if there is any concern about the ability to breathe.

Submit **your** medical emergency story or experience, and find recommended website links at: www.saveyourlifebook.com

Chapter 8

Bleeding

If you see a person bleeding heavily, or you think they might be bleeding internally, call 9-1-1 immediately.

If possible, before you try to stop severe bleeding, wash your hands and put on synthetic gloves. If you don't have synthetic gloves, you can use clean freezer bags to cover your hands.

If there is a deep cut in the abdomen and internal organs are pushing out of the wound, don't try to push them back into place; just cover the wound with a dressing or a clean cloth.

Seven Ways to Help

Call 9-1-1. Then Do the Following Seven Things:

1. Lie the person down and cover them to prevent loss of body heat.

2. If possible, position the person's head slightly lower than their trunk or lift the legs to reduce the risk of fainting. Then elevate the site of the bleeding.

3. Remove any obvious dirt or debris from the wound. *Use gloves or a clean plastic bag to cover your hands.*

4. Apply pressure directly on the wound until the bleeding stops.

5. Use a sterile bandage or clean cloth and continue applying pressure for at least 20 minutes.

6. Maintain pressure by binding the wound tightly with a bandage (or a piece of clean cloth) and adhesive tape. Use your hands if nothing else is available.

7. Squeeze a main artery, if necessary. If the bleeding doesn't stop with direct pressure, apply pressure to the artery delivering blood to the area of the wound.

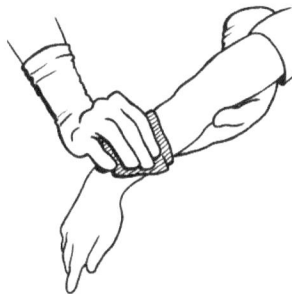

- The places to apply pressure on the arm are on the inside of the arm just above the elbow and just below the armpit.

- The places to apply pressure on the leg are just behind the knee and in the groin.

- Squeeze the main artery in these areas against the bone. Keep your fingers flat. With your other hand, continue to keep pressure on the wound itself.

Five Things Not Do

1. Never probe the wound or attempt to clean it. *Your main concern is to stop the bleeding.*

2. Never remove any large or deeply embedded objects. It could make things worse.

3. Don't look to see if the bleeding has stopped. Just keep pressing the wound.

4. Do not remove the gauze or bandage. If the bleeding continues and seeps through it or other material, just add more absorbent material to what is already there.

5. Don't move the injured body part once the bleeding has stopped, or remove the bandages.[15]

---

[15] Medline Plus, A service of the U.S. National Library of Medicine
National Institutes of Health

Recognizing Internal Bleeding

Call 9-1-1 if you see these signs of internal bleeding:

- Abdominal tenderness, possibly along with very tight abdominal muscles

- Bleeding from the ears, nose, rectum, vagina or other body cavities

- Bruising on neck, chest, abdomen or side between ribs and hip)

- Fractures

- Shock, indicated by weakness, anxiety, thirst or skin that is cool to the touch

- Vomiting or coughing up blood

- Wounds that have penetrated the skull, chest or abdomen

Chapter 9

Burns

Burns are common. More than 500,000[16] people in the United States are treated for burns and 3,000 to 4,000 people die from severe burns each year.[17] Older people and young children are most at risk.

What would you do if you saw someone on fire?

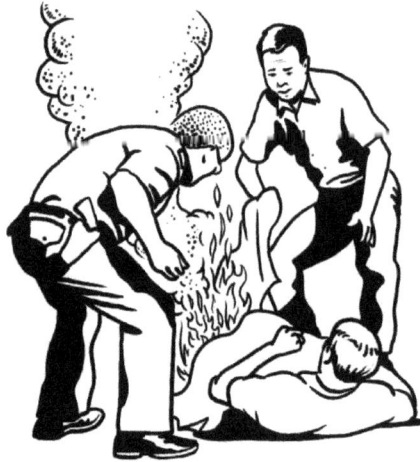

[16] National Hospital Ambulatory Medical Care Survey; National Ambulatory Medical Care Survey; Medical Expenditure Panel; CPSC/NEISS (National Electronic Injury Surveillance System), (2000-2004 data).

[17] National Fire Protection Association (2005); American Burn Association National Burn Repository (2005 report); US Vital Statistics (2004).

Stop, Drop, and Roll

Remember, if someone is on fire, tell them: "Do not run!" Running will fan the flames. Tell them to **stop** running or walking, **drop** to the ground, and **roll** on the ground to put out the flames. If you have a thick jacket or blanket, use it to wrap the person and smother the flames, then gently douse the person with cool water.

Submit *your* medical emergency story or experience, and find recommended website links at: www.saveyourlifebook.com

This is a story of what happened when I was with my dad many years ago.

Man on Fire

Once when I was a boy, I was out to eat with my family. As we walked out of the restaurant, we saw a man working under the hood of his car while smoking a cigarette. Suddenly, he burst into flames and began to run, making the fire worse. We yelled at him to stop running, but he would not stop.

It was winter, and I was wearing a thick Army Navy jacket.

My father and I ran after him. My father was a former football player and marine. He tackled the man as I threw my coat on him and the fire was put out. There were no cell phones then and we went back into the restaurant and called 9-1-1. It all happened very fast. –MS

Three Types of Burns

Doctors describe burns by their severity:

- **First-degree** burns affect only the outer layer of the skin. They cause pain, redness, and swelling.

- **Second-degree** burns affect both the outer and middle layer of skin. They cause blistering in addition to pain and redness, and swelling.

- **Third-degree** burns are deeper and penetrate all three skin layers. These burns make the skin appear white or blackened. Charred skin may be numb because the nerves have been destroyed. If the skin near a third-degree burn has a second-degree burn, it can be extremely painful.

Burns can easily become infected if not treated quickly and properly.

When to Call 9-1-1 for Burns

- The burn is caused by chemicals or electricity.

- The burn is deep (goes through all layers of the skin).

- The burn is on the face, hands, feet or genitalia (groin).

- The burn is the size of your palm or larger, or you are unsure of the burn's severity.

- The person inhaled smoke.

- The person shows signs of shock, (palo, olammy skin; weakness; bluish lips and finger nails).

- You know, or think, someone burned the person on purpose.

When a person suffers any type of burn, first call 9-1-1, then:

- Make sure the person isn't touching any smoldering materials.

- Gently cool the burned area with cool running water **(not ice cold)** until the ambulance arrives. Skin continues to burn even after the fire is extinguished. Cooling the burned area can stop shallow burns from becoming deeper.[18]

- Separate burned fingers or toes with a dry, sterile, non-adhesive dressing between them.

- Cover the burn with a cool, moist, sterile bandage or clean cloth, if available. Sheets work best for large burns.

- Make sure the person is breathing. If breathing has stopped or if the person's airway is blocked, open the airways. If necessary, begin hands only CPR (see pages 132-133).

- Elevate the burned body part above the level of the heart. Protect the burn area from pressure and friction.

- Lay the person flat to prevent shock. Elevate their feet about 12 inches, and cover the person with a clean cloth.

---

[18] http://www.bt.cdc.gov/masscasualties/burns.asp

Seven Things Not to Do After a Burn[19]

1. Don't breathe, blow, or cough on the burn. It can cause infection.

2. Don't give the person anything by mouth if there is a severe burn.

3. Don't pop blisters or remove dead skin.

4. Don't place a pillow under the person's head if there is an airways burn; this can close the airways.

5. Don't use icy cold water and ice cubes. This could damage burned skin further.

6. Never place the person in the shock position (with feet 12 inches higher than the head) if you suspect the person has a head, neck, back, or leg injury, or if it makes the person uncomfortable.

7. Don't put cream, ointment, butter, medications, oil spray, or any household remedy on a severe burn. They trap heat and cause burns to continue simmering instead of cooling.

---

[19] "Burns: Medline Plus Medical Encyclopedia." National Library of Medicine - National Institutes of Health. Web. 17 Dec. 2010.

Children under age four and adults over age 60 have a higher chance of complications and death from severe burns.

Call a doctor immediately if the person has any of the following signs of infection:

- Increased pain, redness, swelling, drainage or pus from the burn

- Swollen lymph nodes

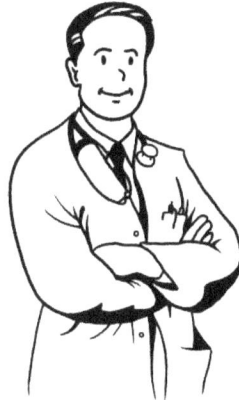

- Red streaks spreading from the burn

- Fever

In addition to infection, dehydration is a serious potential complication of burns. Call a doctor immediately if you notice any of these four signs of dehydration.

Four Ds of dehydration:

1. **Dry mouth** (extreme thirst)
2. **Dry skin**
3. **Dizziness** or lightheadedness
4. **Decreased** urination

Children, elderly, or anyone with a weakened Immune system, such as HIV/AIDS should be seen at once if they have burns. This also applies to anyone with cancer, kidney disease, or who is receiving chemotherapy.

Chapter 10

Choking

Choking occurs when a person's throat (airway) is blocked. There is a real likelihood of death or brain damage if the blockage is not quickly removed.

Although choking is most often caused by food or other objects stuck in the throat, **never** stick your fingers into a choking person's mouth. There is a good possibility you will be bitten and not be able to remove whatever is stuck in their throat.

Although many restaurants now have special tongs to help get food out of a choking person's throat, it is good to know how to perform the Heimlich maneuver. It's easy, and you don't have to be a doctor to do it.

How to Do the Heimlich Maneuver

If the victim is sitting or standing, follow these steps [20]

1. Make a fist with your hand with the thumb and index finger forming a knob. Press this knob directly against the patient's stomach, above the navel but below the sternum or breastbone.

2. With your free hand, reach around and grab your fist. Press the fist up and into the stomach with a sharp thrusting motion. Be sure to make this thrust by bending both elbows, not by "hugging" the choking person. A strong hug can crack ribs.

If the victim is lying face down, follow these steps:

1. Roll the person onto their back.

2. Remember to make sure their chin is pointed up in order to clear the airway.

---

[20] http://www.heimlichinstitute.org/page.php?id=34

3. Place one hand on top of the other with the heel of the lower hand against the victim's stomach, again between their navel and sternum (breast bone).

4. Press into and up against the victim's stomach with a sharp thrusting motion.

For both the standing and lying Heimlich maneuvers, the thrust may be repeated several times, if necessary, until the patient can breathe, and returns to consciousness and normal color.

If the technique does not seem to be working after a few trioo:

Call 9-1-1 immediately

Heimlich Maneuver

1. Lean the person forward slightly and stand behind him or her.

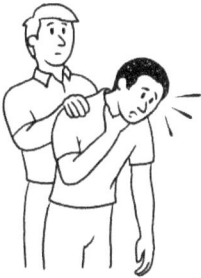

2. Make a fist with one hand.

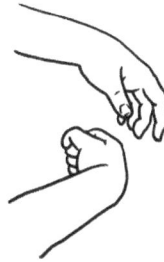

3. Put your arms around the person and grasp your fist with your other hand near the top of the stomach and below the center of the rib cage.

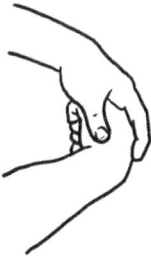

4. Make a quick, hard movement inward and upward.

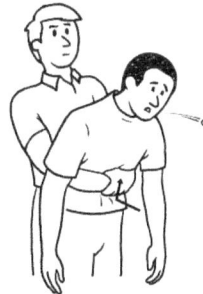

Here is a story that happened to me.

Choking Happens Quickly

As a young doctor, I was with friends at a dinner theatre, enjoying my meal before the show began. Suddenly, a very anxious manager of the restaurant shouted that a woman was choking in the bathroom and if there was a doctor present, please come quickly.

I went into the bathroom and found a middle-aged woman lying on the floor and turning blue. While eating French onion soup she had gasped, and a large piece of the cheese got sucked into her throat and covered her windpipe.

I lifted the woman up to the sitting position, picked her up and performed the Heimlich maneuver. The cheese popped out. In a few minutes, everyone went back to their seats and the dinner show began. –MS

Chapter 11

Diabetes

Most likely, you know someone with diabetes. It affects nearly 18 million people [21] and is a problem of control of blood-sugar levels. When people eat, most of the carbohydrates in their food are broken down into a form of sugar called glucose. Glucose circulates in the blood and is the body's main source of fuel for growth and energy. People with diabetes are not able to regulate their blood-glucose levels.

In order for glucose to be absorbed and used by the cells, a hormone called insulin, produced by the pancreas, must be present. Someone who is diabetic has either too little or no insulin, or their cells do not respond correctly to the insulin that is produced. People with diabetes must take insulin or other medications to regulate their glucose levels and should check their blood glucose levels according to their doctor's recommendations. If blood glucose is not regulated, serious medical problems can occur.

---

[21] http://www.ghsa.net/diabetes-mellitus-symptoms-management-and-prevention

Two potentially life threatening complications of diabetes are:

1. **Diabetic coma,** which occurs when blood glucose levels get too high. This can be caused by eating too much sugar or carbohydrates, not enough insulin, extreme stress, or illness.

2. **Insulin shock**, which occurs when blood glucose levels become too low. This can be caused by too much insulin, or other diabetes medications, not eating enough, excessive alcohol or increased activity.

Recognizing a Diabetic Coma

If a person with diabetes has the following symptoms they may have diabetic coma: **Call 9-1-1** if you suspect diabetic coma.

- Change in the level of consciousness or confusion
- Deep and fast breathing
- Nausea or vomiting
- Unusual drowsiness
- Excessive thirst or a very dry mouth
- Dry or flushed skin
- Sweet or fruity-smelling breath

Saving Someone in Insulin Shock

Too much insulin is dangerous. If blood-glucose levels get too low, a person with diabetes can have an insulin reaction which untreated can lead to insulin shock. **They need sugar immediately.** Give them a small glass of fruit juice, a regular soda (tonic), or something else with sugar such as candy. If they do not feel better in a few minutes or are unconscious or unresponsive, **call 9-1-1 immediately**.

Symptoms of Insulin Shock

- Confusion, change in level of consciousness
- Weakness
- Vision difficulties
- Fast breathing, dizziness
- Fast pulse, sweating
- Headache,
- Unusual hunger
- Numbness in hands or feet

Both diabetic coma and insulin shock can be life-threatening, but insulin shock is an emergency that requires immediate medical attention. People with diabetes often wear a medical alert bracelet so in an emergency, others will know they are diabetic.

If you see someone with that bracelet who is acting strangely or having any of the symptoms listed above, **call 9-1-1 and give them some form of sugar.** Something as simple as a small glass of fruit juice, a half can of regular soda (tonic), or anything else with sugar in it, such as hard candy can save their life!

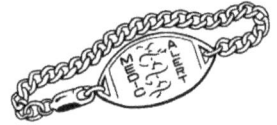

Alert! If you have diabetes:

1. Always keep a small bottle of glucose liquid or glucose tablets with you.

2. When eating out, if you take insulin always remember to take it with you.

3. Check your blood sugar level as prescribed by your doctor.

Chapter 12

Falls and Slips

Each year, one in every three adults age 65 and older falls.[22] [23] Did you know that falls are the major cause of fatal and nonfatal injuries for people 65 and older? 18,000 older adults died from injuries related to falls in 2007 and about 2.1 million were treated in emergency rooms in 2008. The number of deaths and injuries continues to rise each year as the population ages.[24]

Many serious falls happen at home and can be prevented.

---

[22] Hausdorff JM, Rios DA, Edelber HK. Gait variability and fall risk in community–living older adults: a 1–year prospective study. Archives of Physical Medicine and Rehabilitation 2001; 82(8): 1050–6.

[23] Hornbrook MC, Stevens VJ, Wingfield DJ, Hollis JF, Greenlick MR, Ory MG. Preventing falls among community–dwelling older persons: results from a randomized trial. The Gerontologist 1994:34(1):16–23.

[24] http://www.cdc.gov/HomeandRecreationalSafety/Falls/adultfalls.html

Eight Ways to Prevent Falls

1. Clean up spills immediately, especially liquids, grease, or food.

2. Avoid ladders. Keep clothing, dishes, food and other household items in easy-to-reach places.

3. Keep paths clear. Place coffee tables, magazine racks, and plant stands away from high-traffic areas.

4. Keep floors and carpets smooth and securely tacked down. Repair loose, wooden floorboards.

5. Use nonskid floor wax.

6. Use nonskid mats in your bathtub or shower.

7. Keep walkways clear and free of anything you can trip on (boxes, papers, electrical/phone cords, etc).

8. Use double faced tape, tacks, or a slip-resistant backing on loose rugs so you won't trip on them.

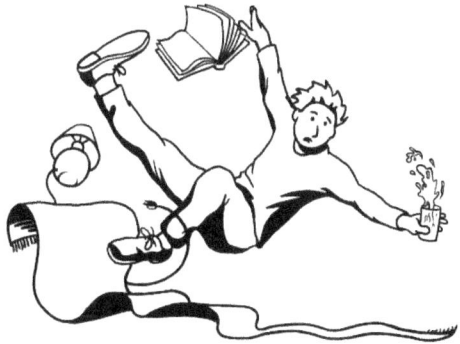

She Slipped and Broke Her Hip

Ella, a spry 80-year-old, wanted to get a bottle of oil from the kitchen cabinet, but couldn't reach it. She decided to climb on a step stool to get the oil. It seemed like a reasonable thing to do.

However, as she was stepping off the stool she dropped the bottle of oil, which was not sealed tightly. When it hit the floor it opened and created a slippery puddle around the stool. Ella thought she could step over it, but ended up slipping and breaking her hip. That caused her to need extensive surgery.

Fortunately, after the operation and several months of physical therapy, Ella recovered and was able to continue living on her own. –SG

If Ella had kept things within easy reach, her accident would not have happened. Step stools or ladders can be very dangerous, especially for seniors.

It is not worth the risk.

Fall Proofing Your Home

People over 65 or younger individuals with physical disabilities can benefit from these additional safeguards for bathrooms, stairs, and improved vision that are easy-to-do and make you and your home safer.[25]

Bathrooms:

- Place a sturdy plastic seat in your shower or tub so you can sit down if needed.

- Buy a hand-held shower nozzle so you can shower sitting down.

- Place grab bars inside and just outside your shower or bathtub.

- Use a raised toilet seat or one with armrests to steady you.

---

[25] http://arthritis.about.com/od/preventionandriskfactors/ht/slipsfalls.htm

Stairs:

- Install light switches at the top and bottom of stairs.

- Install handrails on both sides of stairways.

- Use nonskid treads on bare-wood steps.

- Turn on the lights before going up or down stairs.

Vision:

- Check the prescription for your eyeglasses regularly to maintain your best vision.

- Have plenty of light. Keep a lamp near your bed with a switch that is easy to reach and turn on. Be sure to use it when you get up at night.

- Make clear paths to light switches that aren't near room entrances. If possible have Glow-in-the-dark or illuminated switches.

- Place a night-light in your bedroom, bathrooms, and hallways.

- Store flashlights in easy-to-find places in case of power outages.

For more suggestions on how to make your house safer, speak with your doctor and ask for a referral to an occupational therapist.

Alone Without Help

A friend of my mother lived alone. She stepped out of her front door and slipped in a narrow entrance porch where she could not be seen from the outside.

Her leg was broken but she didn't have a cell phone with her or a medical alert device. She waited in pain for over 12 hours to be found. –MS

Chapter 13

Head Injuries

Do you remember the actress Natasha Richardson who hit her head while skiing on a beginner slope in 2009? At the time, she seemed to be fine. Unfortunately, a few hours later she died from complications of her fall. Even the most seemingly minor head injuries can be fatal.

Be safe...Call 9-1-1.

Head injuries cause approximately 52,000 deaths, and 275,000 hospitalizations in the US each year,[26] and over 1.3 million people require emergency room treatment. Never ignore a head injury.

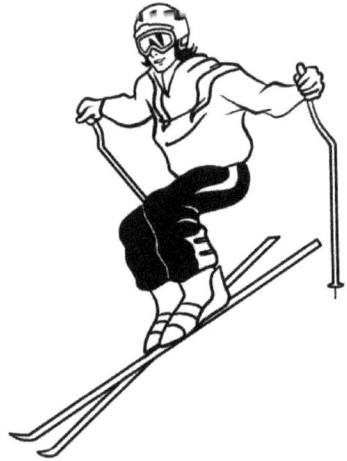

---

[26] http://www.cdc.gov/TraumaticBrainInjury/statistics.html

How to Prevent Head Injuries

Can you lower your risk of a head injury?

Yes! You can protect yourself by always wearing an approved helmet for sports like skiing, biking, and rollerblading.

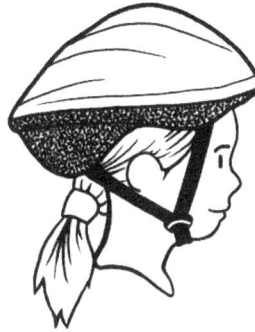

The following information will help you determine if and when to seek medical care or call 9-1-1. However, if you have any question or concerns about a head injury always contact a physician and seek medical advice.

Symptoms of Head Injuries

Call 9-1-1 after a head injury if any of the following symptoms are, or were, present:

- A headache or "pressure" in their head

- Balance problems or dizziness

- Bleeding

- Blood or clear fluid from their mouth, ears or nose

- Failure to recall events either *after* or *prior* to a hit or fall

- Concentration difficulty, memory problems, or confusion

- A feeling of depression or not "feeling right"

- Double or blurry vision

- A sluggish feeling; a sense of feeling foggy or groggy

- Impaired hearing, smell, taste, or vision

- Inability to move one or more limbs

- Irritability (especially in children), personality changes, or unusual behavior

- Loss of consciousness, even briefly

- Nausea or vomiting

- Pain
- Problem focusing eyes normally
- Seizures
- Sensitivity to light or noise
- Trouble breathing or no breathing

Sometimes symptoms improve and then suddenly get worse. Call 9-1-1 if this happens or there are other signs that worry you or the person with the head injury

Call 9-1-1 if a child receives a head injury and has any of the symptoms listed above or *any of these three conditions*:[27]

1. Does not stop crying and cannot be comforted

2. Refuses to nurse or eat

3. Appears confused or has memory loss

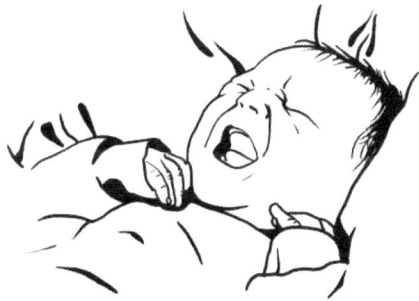

---

[27] http://www.mayoclinic.com/health/traumatic-brain-injury/DS00552/DSECTION=symptoms

After a Head Injury

- Do not allow someone to drink alcohol within 48 hours.

- Do not move the person unless absolutely necessary. (Moving an injured person can make the problem worse. This is especially important for an injured child who should not be picked up.)

- Do not remove a helmet if you suspect a serious head injury.

- Do not remove any object sticking out of a wound.

- Do not shake the injured person if he or she seems dazed.

- Do not wash a head wound that is deep or bleeding a lot.

If an accident happens, call 9-1-1 before you do anything to a person who has fallen. Tell the operator where you are, what happened, and the person's symptoms. Stay on the phone and follow the operator's instructions. Try to stay calm and let the injured person know help is on the way.

A Flash by the Window and a Thud

I was sitting in the living room, waiting for the TV service man to finish repairing the roof antenna, when suddenly something flashed by the window, followed by an awful thud. I ran out and found the young technician lying on the icy ground. He had fallen off the roof. I felt a moment of panic, but immediately called 9-1-1 on my cell phone.

The operator told me to stay on the line, not to move the man, but to cover him and keep him warm. I sat beside him for what seemed like an eternity, told him help was on the way and he'd be all right. Finally, the ambulance and police arrived and took him to the hospital.

I later learned that, thankfully, his injuries were not serious. –SG

Chapter 14

Meningitis

Meningitis is an inflammation of the covering that surrounds the brain and the spinal cord. It can be caused either by virus or bacteria.

Bacterial meningitis can cause problems such as brain damage, hearing loss, and learning difficulties. It can also cause death within just a few hours of the onset of symptoms.

Viral meningitis is usually not as severe as bacterial meningitis. However, it is difficult to tell the difference without lab tests, so it is extremely important to seek medical care at once if meningitis is suspected.

There is a vaccination for some types of bacterial meningitis. Ask your doctor if you or members of your family should be vaccinated.

Symptoms of Meningitis

Call 9-1-1 if there is a sudden onset of one, or any, of these symptoms:

- A sensitivity to bright light

- A stiff neck

- High fever

- Nausea and vomiting

- One pupil (the black part in the middle of the eye) is larger than the other

- Severe headache that does not go away

- Sleepiness or trouble waking up

Infant's symptoms of meningitis may also include: [28]

- Irritability

- Listlessness

- Drowsiness

- Loss of appetite or poor feeding

- Jaundice (a yellowish skin tone)

---

[28] http://kidshealth.org/parent/infections/lung/meningitis.html

Sudden Illness Can Be a Medical Emergency

When I was about five years old, my mother suddenly got very ill. She had a terrible headache, started to vomit, and could not move her head. She was very tired and had a high fever. We called an ambulance. The driver and another man came in and quickly took my mother out on a stretcher. I stood at the screen door and watched them roll my mother into the back of the ambulance and close the door behind her.

Before they left, the driver came back to the front door and told me my mother had meningitis. He said she was going to the hospital and that I could not visit her because I might catch it. He told me that she was very sick and I might not see her again. I stood at the front door as they drove away with my mother.

She's now 86, but I have never forgotten that day. —MS

Chapter 15

Poisoning

Did you know that most accidental poisonings are due to medicines or household chemicals, and that adults between the ages of 34 and 56 are more likely to die from poisonings than from motor vehicle accidents?[29]

Most people know that poison can make them very sick or kill them if they eat, breathe, inject, or even touch enough of it. They also know that some poisons work quickly, while others may take longer to seriously affect or kill them, but they often don't know the signs of poisoning or what to do.

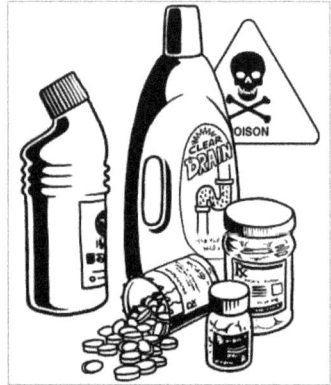

Many people do not know that mixing medications or taking someone else's medication can cause serious problems or death. Do not take someone else's medication even if they

---

29 http://www.cdc.gov/HomeandRecreationalSafety/Poisoning/index.html

have "similar" symptoms. Always speak with your doctor before mixing or taking any medication.

This section will tell you how to prevent accidental poisoning, how to recognize the symptoms of it, and what you should do (or not do) if you think someone has been poisoned.

Nine Ways to Help Prevent Accidental Poisoning From Medications

1. Call your pharmacist or doctor if not sure when or how to take medication.

2. Always store medicines out of a child's reach and use childproof caps.

3. Make sure all medicines and chemicals are labeled correctly.

4. Always take or give medicines in a lighted room to be sure it's the right amount of the right medicine.

5. Do not keep medicines after their expiration date or once you have been told to stop taking them.

6. Do not keep medicines with no expiration date if they are more than a year old.

7. Do not remove medicine labels from containers. Without the label, you might take the wrong medicine.

8. Do not take or give medicine if you cannot read the label.

9. Never take or give medicine meant for someone else. It can cause serious illness or death.

Five Ways to Help Prevent Accidental Chemical Poisoning

1. Always read labels before handling chemicals such as pesticides, cleaning fluids, and solvents. Follow the instructions on the label.

2. Always store poisonous products away from children.

3. Do not remove chemicals from their original container.

4. Never store household chemicals in soda bottles or other safe-looking containers. Children, and even adults, may be fooled into thinking it's safe to eat or drink.

5. Never store poisonous items in areas where food or beverages are kept.

Signs of Poisoning

Call 9-1-1 if you see signs of poisoning, such as:

- Breath that smells like chemicals, such as gasoline or paint thinner

- Burns or redness around the mouth and lips, which can result from drinking certain poisons

- Burns, stains, and odors on the person, their clothes, or the furniture, floor, rugs, or other objects nearby

- Empty medication bottles or scattered pills

- Vomiting, difficulty breathing, sleepiness, confusion, or other unexpected signs

Call 9-1-1 immediately if the person is:

- Drowsy or unconscious

- Having difficulty breathing or has stopped breathing

- Having seizures

- Uncontrollably restless or agitated

Even if the person doesn't have any of these symptoms, but you still believe they have taken a poisonous substance, call:

The U.S. Poison Control Center

1-800-222-1222

Tell the operator at the Poison Control Center the person's symptoms and, if possible, what and how much they took, and when they took it.

If you are told to go to the hospital take the poison container (or any pill bottles) with you.

Care For a Poison Victim Until EMTs Arrive

- When the person has been exposed to poisonous fumes, such as gas or carbon monoxide, get them into fresh air immediately. If you cannot move them, open doors and windows.

- If the person swallowed poison, remove anything remaining in their mouth.

- When the suspected poison is a household cleaner or other chemical, read the label and follow instructions for accidental poisoning.

- If the poison came in contact with the person's eyes or skin, flush the eyes or skin with cool or lukewarm water. If you can, use a shower for 20 minutes or until help arrives.

- If the poison spilled on the person's clothing, remove the clothing.

Call the US Poison Control Center if:

- You cannot identify the poison

- The substance taken was a medication

- There are no instructions regarding the substance taken

- You need advice regarding a toxic substance

Follow the treatment directions given to you by the Poison Control Center.

Add the US Poison Control Center's number to all your mobile phones (1-800-222-1222) to save valuable time in case of a poisoning.

Poisoning can look like many other conditions. It can cause seizures, stroke symptoms, or make a person look like they are drunk or a diabetic with a very low blood sugar.[30] If you think it is even possible that a person has been poisoned, call 9-1-1.

---

[30] http://www.mayoclinic.com/health/first-aid-poisoning/FA00029

Do not give a victim anything before you check with the U.S. Poison Control Center at (**1-800-222-1222**) because you could make their condition worse.

Note: Do not try to make the person vomit or give them ipecac syrup, which causes vomiting. In fact, the American Academy of Pediatrics advises not having ipecac in the home because it can do more harm than good.[31]

Submit *your* medical emergency story or experience, and find recommended website links at: www.saveyourlifebook.com

---

[31] http://www.mayoclinic.com/health/first-aid-poisoning/FA00029

Recognizing Food Poisoning

Bacteria that you cannot see, smell or taste can cause food poisoning. Each year, food poisoning affects approximately 76 million Americans, causing up to 5,000 deaths and 325,000 hospitalizations.[32] While it generally lasts only about 48 hours, there can be complications that require immediate medical care.

Eight Common Symptoms of Food Poisoning

1. Abdominal cramping
2. Bloody stools
3. Chills
4. Diarrhea
5. Fever
6. Nausea
7. Vomiting
8. Dehydration

---

[32] http://www.cdc.gov/ncidod/eid/vol5no5/mead.htm

Call 9-1-1 if any of the following eight symptoms occur:

1. Swelling in one or more joints or a rash on the skin

2. Sharp or cramping pains that last for over ten to fifteen minutes

3. Swollen stomach or abdomen

4. Problems with breathing, speaking, or swallowing

5. Decreased urination or dark-colored urine

6. Vomiting blood or bloody bowel movements

7. Fainting, dizziness, lightheadedness, or vision problems

8. Yellow skin and/or eyes

If you, or the person who is ill, feel it's an emergency, call 9-1-1.

Even if a victim of food poisoning is not showing serious symptoms, you should seek medical care if the following conditions are observed:

- Nausea, vomiting, or diarrhea lasts more than two days, even though the person is drinking large amounts of fluid.

- Other family members or friends who ate the same food also are sick.

- Symptoms begin after recent foreign travel.

- The ill person cannot take prescribed medications because of vomiting.

- The ill person is less than three years old.

- The person has a disease or illness that weakens their immune system, such as HIV/AIDS, cancer, or kidney disease, or they're undergoing chemotherapy.

- The person has any nervous system symptoms, such as slurred speech, muscle weakness, double vision, or difficulty swallowing.

- There are abdominal symptoms and low-grade fever.

There are a few simple steps you can take to prevent food poisoning when shopping for, storing, and preparing food.

Safe Shopping

Buy cold foods as the last item on your shopping trip. Bring them home quickly to prevent bacteria from growing. When it's very hot outside, bring a cooler with ice to keep things cold.

Remember the following three things:

1. Do not buy foods past their "sell-by" or expiration dates.

2. When shopping, keep raw meat and poultry separate from other foods.

3. Never buy torn or leaking packages.

Safe Food Storage

Once you bring food home, there are a few simple things you can do to keep your food safely stored:

- Check the temperature of your refrigerator. To slow bacterial growth, the food section should be at 40°F, the freezer at 0°F.

- Cook or freeze fresh poultry, fish, ground meats, and variety meats within two days.

- Unload perishable foods first and refrigerate them immediately. Place raw meat, fish, or poultry in the coldest section of your refrigerator.

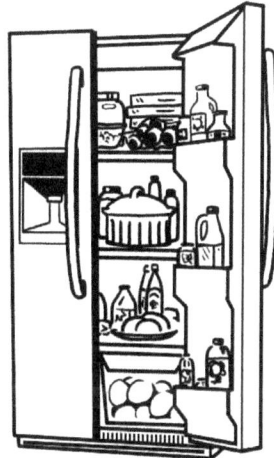

Safe Food Preparation

Clean food preparation surfaces are just as important to food safety as good storage. Keep in mind the following as you work with food in your kitchen:

- Wash hands before and after handling raw meat and poultry.

- Keep raw meat, fish, poultry, and their juices away from other food.

- After cutting raw meats, wash your hands, the cutting board, the counter tops and the knife with hot, soapy water.

- Marinate meat and poultry in a covered dish in the refrigerator and discard any uncooked or unused marinade.

- Clean cutting boards often by washing with a solution of one teaspoon chlorine bleach mixed with four cups of water.

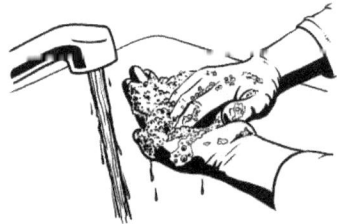

Chapter 16

Seizures

Would you know what to do if you saw someone having a seizure? Here's what one boy did.

Eleven-Year-Old Saves Mom

When eleven-year-old Ethan found his mother, who was six months pregnant, having a violent seizure on Thanksgiving eve, he knew exactly what to do. Ethan said he learned about the condition in a medical book he found around the house. He remembered its first aid instructions and knew to call 9-1-1. After calling 9-1-1, he rolled his mother onto her stomach to keep her from choking, dressed his younger siblings, and waited until help arrived.

Ethan's quick actions saved his mother's life and possibly the life of her unborn baby.[33]

---

33 "Dorchester Boy Took Charge to save Mother - The Boston Globe." Boston.com. Web. 30 Dec. 2010. <http://www.boston.com/news /local / Massachusetts/articles/2010/12/27/ Dorchester_boy_took_charge_to_save his mother

What are Seizures?

Seizures (also called convulsions) are caused by an uncontrolled discharge of electricity in the brain. They can be triggered by reactions to medicines, high fevers, head injuries and certain diseases.

Nearly ten percent of Americans have a seizure at some point in their lives[34] and they can happen at any age. Most seizures last from 30 seconds to 2 minutes and do not cause lasting harm,[35] especially in people who have recurring seizures due to epilepsy. However, there are times when a seizure could indicate a life-threatening emergency.

Having a strange feeling in your stomach can be a sign of a fleeting seizure. Other signs include blanking out for a few seconds or jerking movements in your arm, leg or your body. These should be discussed with a doctor.

---

[34] "Epilepsy Foundation-Epilepsy and Seizure Statistics." *Epilepsy Foundation-Epilepsy Foundation-trusted, Reliable Information for People with Seizures, and Their Caregivers*. Web. 13 Jan. 2011. <http://www.epilepsyfoundation.org/about/statistics.cfm>.

[35] http://www.epilepsyfoundation.org/about/firstaid/index.cfm

Here is a list of seizure symptoms.[36] Some people may have other symptoms that are not listed. Let you physician know if you have any of these symptoms.

Nine Common Seizure Symptoms

1. Blacking out, falling down, shaking

2. Loss of consciousness, confusion

3. Deafness/ strange sounds

4. Electric shock feeling

5. Unusual smell

6. Spacing out

7. Out-of-body experience

8. Visual loss or blurring

9. Fear/panic

---

[36] "Symptoms of a Seizure | Epilepsy.com." *Epilepsy and Seizure Information for Patients and Health Professionals | Epilepsy.com*. Web. 30 Dec. 2010. <http://www.epilepsy .com/101 / Ep101_symptom>.

There may be different feelings or behaviors that occur at the beginning of a seizure, during it, or at the end. These symptoms may be an alert that a seizure is about to begin or can be part of the seizure itself. Sometimes seizures occur without warning symptoms.

Additional Seizure Symptoms

- Chewing movements, drooling

- Convulsion

- Difficulty talking

- Eyelid fluttering, eyes rolling up

- Foot stomping, hand waving

- Inability to move

- Incontinence

- Lip smacking, teeth clenching/grinding

- Making involuntary sounds

- Staring

- Stiffening, breathing difficulty

- Swallowing, tongue biting

- Sweating

- Tremors, twitching movements

- Heart racing

Seven Reasons To Call 9-1-1 For a Seizure[37]

1. It is a first-time seizure

2. The seizure does not stop within a few minutes.

3. Confusion, after the seizure, lasts for more than 10-15 minutes.

4. The person is not responsive after a seizure.

5. There is a breathing problem after the seizure.

6. There has been an injury during the seizure.

7. There is a meaningful change in the type of seizure from the ones the person has had before.

---

37 http://www.emedicinehealth.com/seizures_emergencies/article _em.htm# Seizures %20
Emergencies%20Overview

Possible Feelings after a Seizure

- Memory loss, confusion

- Difficulty writing

- Depression and sadness or fear

- Frustration, shame/embarrassment

- Injuries, bruising, pain

- Difficulty talking

- Desire to sleep

- Exhaustion, weakness

- Headache, nausea

- Thirst

- Urge to urinate/defecate

First Aid For Seizures

Nine Things to Do

1. Time the seizure with your watch and tell first responders how long it lasted.

2. Make sure there is nothing hard or sharp around the person having a seizure.

3. Loosen ties or anything around the neck.

4. Keep calm and reassure people who are nearby.

5. Put something flat and soft, like a folded jacket, under the person's head.

6. Turn the person gently onto one side to help keep the airway clear.

7. If a child is having a seizure, due to a high fever, wait until the seizure stops, and then lower their temperature by sponging their body with room temperature water.

8. Be reassuring as consciousness returns.

9. Stay with the person until the seizure ends naturally

If a person seems confused or unable to get home call 9-1-1.

Seven Things Not to Do During a Seizure

1. Never try to hold the person down or try to stop his or her movements.

2. Do not try to force the mouth open with any hard implement or with fingers. A person having a seizure **CANNOT** swallow his tongue (trying to hold the tongue down can injure teeth or the jaw).

3. Do not throw water on their face.

4. Do not use ice.

5. Do not attempt artificial respiration unless the person is not breathing after the seizure has stopped.

6. Never put a child having a seizure in a bathtub.

7. Do not use rubbing alcohol.

Ten Other Reasons to Call 9-1-1 for Seizures

If the person is or has:

1. Diabetes or hypoglycemia

2. Heat exhaustion

3. Pregnant

4. Been poisoned

5. A high fever

6. A brain infection

7. Electric shock

8. Head injuries

9. Symptoms of meningitis, flu, or chicken pox

10. Been unresponsive or confused

An uncomplicated seizure in someone with epilepsy is not a medical emergency. It usually stops naturally after a few minutes. The average person who has an epileptic seizure is able to continue normally after a rest period and may need only limited help (or no help at all) in getting home. Call 9-1-1 if the person who has had the seizure does not seem better and able to manage on their own after a few minutes.[38]

---

[38] "Epilepsy Foundation-First Aid for Seizures." *Epilepsy Foundation-Epilepsy Foundation-trusted, Reliable Information for People with Seizures, and Their Caregivers*. Web. 30 Dec. 2010. <http://www.epilepsyfoundation.org/about/firstaid/>.

Chapter 17

Additional Information

How to Perform "Hands Only" CPR on Adults

If you see an adult suddenly collapse, call 9-1-1 immediately. Then, if the person has not started breathing normally, coughing or moving do the following:[39]

- Place the heel of one hand on the center of the chest.

- Place the heel of the other hand on top of the first hand, lacing fingers together.

- Keep your arms straight; position your shoulders directly over your hands.

- Push hard. Push fast.

- Compress the chest at least two inches.

- Compress at least 100 times per minute.

- Let the chest rise completely before pushing down again, then continue chest compressions.

---

[39] http://handsonlycpr.org/

Do Not Stop Until

- You see an obvious sign of life.

- Another trained person arrives and takes over.

- EMS personnel arrive.

- An AED (Automated External Defibrillator) is ready to use.

Don't be afraid of hurting the person. This action can make the difference of whether or not the person lives or dies.

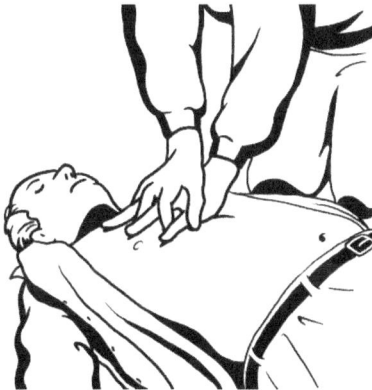

This type of CPR should ***not*** be done on infants or children.

If You Call 9-1-1 by Accident

Stay on the line and say the call was a mistake. That lets the dispatcher know a police officer is not needed.

Ten Reasons Not To Dial 9-1-1

1. As a joke

2. To ask a non-emergency question

3. If there's property damage, but the suspects have left the scene (Call the local police department)

4. To complain about things, such as a dog barking or loud music

5. To get a cat out of a tree (For help with animals, call your local non-emergency number)

6. To make sure the service works

7. To teach someone how to use 9-1-1

8. If there is a motor vehicle accident with no injuries

9. If there's been a theft from a vehicle

10. If you're angry because your kid won't stop playing video games

Medical Alert Devices

Many older adults and people with disabilities who live by themselves can't get up when they fall. They end up lying on the floor for long periods of time, even when family or friends check in on them regularly. These situations might be avoided if the person wears some type of medical alert device, which can summon help with just the push of a button. Some systems can actually detect when a fall occurs and summon help automatically.

Systems come in different forms, including bracelets, necklaces, and pendants. If you insist on not having a medical alert device, at the very least, carry a cell phone with you at all times.

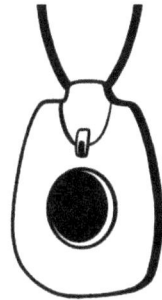

Getting Non-Emergency Help

Up to 40% of 9-1-1 calls are not emergencies. If it's *not* an emergency don't call 9-1-1. Calling unnecessarily can prevent real emergencies from receiving care quickly. It could be **you** or a **loved one** who has to wait because of a false emergency call.

In many cities in the United States and Canada, you can **call 3-1-1** for information and assistance for all non-emergency city services. This service is available 24 hours per day in multiple languages. You can also access 3-1-1 online.

Emergency Numbers Worldwide

If you will be traveling outside the United States, look up the official emergency telephone numbers for each country you plan to visit, and enter them in the cell phone you will be using.

Make sure you have a cell phone that works in the countries you visit, and call your cell phone provider to arrange for phone service in those countries.

Some countries use different emergency numbers for an ambulance, the fire department or police department.

Also, when you are traveling, be sure to bring a copy of your medical history and M.A.D. list with you. They will provide vital information if you have a medical emergency.

For a link to a website with a full alphabetical list of worldwide emergency numbers go to: www.saveyourlifebook.com

Digital Health Reports

Your medical information can now be stored in a wallet sized-card that doctors can easily hook up to a computer. There are several companies that provide wallet-sized flash drives that can contain your vital medical information.

Some hospitals and doctors are also now providing digital backups of your medical records on small devices which you can keep in your purse, pocket or on a key chain.

Ask your doctor or hospital if they offer backups of your medical records. In a medical emergency such devices can save vital time and provide critical information that might help save your life.

Submit *your* medical emergency story or experience, and find recommended website links at: www.saveyourlifebook.com

Medical Expenses

Medical emergencies often lead to a financial emergency. This is true for people both with and without insurance. A study showed that medical expenses cause 62% of all personal bankruptcies.[40] Of these bankruptcies, 78% involved people who had some form of health insurance.

While this book isn't about the cost of medical care, there are a few important things people need to know:

1. When you charge your medical bills with your credit card, it changes your medical debt into a consumer debt. That can lead to penalties and fees if you are late in paying.

2. Your best option is to talk directly with your hospital or provider and negotiate a payment plan. They will usually agree to let you pay over time, rather than all at once. You may also be able to negotiate a

---

[40] "Study Links Medical Costs and Personal Bankruptcy - Business Week." *Business Week - Business News, Stock Market & Financial Advice*. Web. 15 Dec. 2010.

payment plan that is interest free or without penalties or additional fees for a late payment. It's possible you may even have your bill reduced.

3. Before you travel abroad, be sure to read the emergency medical services section of your health insurance policy. Find out if you're covered outside the U.S. for emergency medical care and flight coverage, such as Medevac, should you need to be flown back to the states. If you're not, consider travel insurance, which is relatively inexpensive.

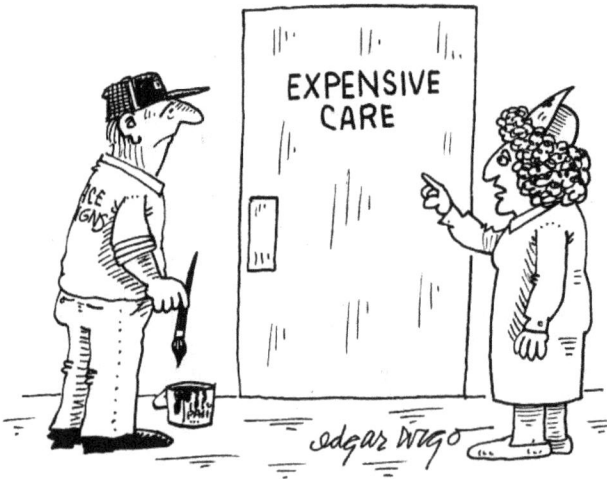

" I HATE TO TELL YOU THIS, BUT THAT SHOULD BE *INTENSIVE* CARE. "

My Emergency Call List

Fill out in pencil, so you can make changes easily

Name: _____

Relationship: _____

Phone Number: _____

Name: _____

Relationship: _____

Phone Number: _____

Name: _____

Relationship: _____

Phone Number: _____

Name: _____

Relationship: _____

Phone Number: _____

My Mad List

Your personalized Medications, Allergies, Doctors (MAD) list includes the following information:

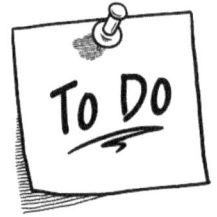

- **Medications**...List the name and dosage of all the medications you take. Be sure to list herbal, organic, and any over-the-counter products you take. Also, include a list of any implanted medical devices you may have, such as a pacemaker.

- **Allergies**...List allergies to any foods or medications you take.

- **Doctors**...List names and phone numbers of your doctors.

My Medications

Medication:
Dosage:
Frequency:
Medication:
Dosage:
Frequency:
Medication:
Dosage:
Frequency:
Medication:
Dosage:
Frequency:
Medication:
Dosage:
Frequency:

Additional Medications

Medication:	
Dosage:	
Frequency:	
Medication:	
Dosage:	
Frequency:	
Medication:	
Dosage:	
Frequency:	
Medication:	
Dosage:	
Frequency:	
Medication:	
Dosage:	
Frequency:	

Additional Medications

Medication:	
Dosage:	
Frequency:	
Medication:	
Dosage:	
Frequency:	
Medication:	
Dosage:	
Frequency:	
Medication:	
Dosage:	
Frequency:	
Medication:	
Dosage:	
Frequency:	

Food Allergies

_____

_____

_____

_____

_____

_____

_____

_____

_____

_____

_____

_____

_____

_____

Other Allergies

My Doctors

List your primary care doctor first.

Name: _____

Specialty: _____

Phone Number: _____

Name: _____

Specialty: _____

Phone Number: _____

Name: _____

Specialty: _____

Phone Number: _____

Name: _____

Specialty: _____

Phone Number: _____

Name: _____

Specialty: _____

Phone Number: _____

Additional Doctors

Name: _____

Specialty: _____

Phone Number: _____

Name: _____

Specialty: _____

Phone Number: _____

Name: _____

Specialty: _____

Phone Number: _____

Name: _____

Specialty: _____

Phone Number: _____

Name: _____

Specialty: _____

Phone Number: _____

Ten Items Someone Hospitalized Might Like

1. Bathrobe

2. Slippers

3. Socks

4. Books, favorite magazines

5. Notepad and pen

6. Glasses

7. Electric toothbrush

8. Razor (men often like to have their own razor)

9. Hairbrush

10. Make-up (women often find it gives them a lift to have a bit of make-up)

Nine Things You May Need If Hospitalized

1. List of phone numbers so family and friends can be called

2. Contact phone number for your place of work

3. Arrangements for pet care, including the pet's name, and where its food is kept

4. Arrangement to have your mail and newspaper picked up or held

5. Location of important bills that will need to be paid

6. Location of insurance papers

7. Instructions on how to set house alarm including the name and phone number of the alarm company and your security code

8. Contact number for your attorney and location of your living will and health care proxy

9. Location of your appointment book

Additional Information

About the Authors

Shelly Glazier, M.Ed., LMFT has taught courses on Medical Emergency Awareness in the Boston area including Brandeis University's BOLLI (adult education) Program. Mrs. Glazier is a licensed marriage and family therapist. She also managed a pediatric practice and worked as a medical administrator for Boston Children's Hospital Pediatric Medical Association.

Mache Seibel, M.D. spent nearly 20 years on the Harvard Medical School faculty and has won multiple national awards for patient education, research, medical writing, and music composition, and the *Distinguished Alumnus Award* from the University of Texas Medical Branch. Dr. Seibel is a professor at the University of Massachusetts Medical School.

For more information visit www.DoctorSeibel.com

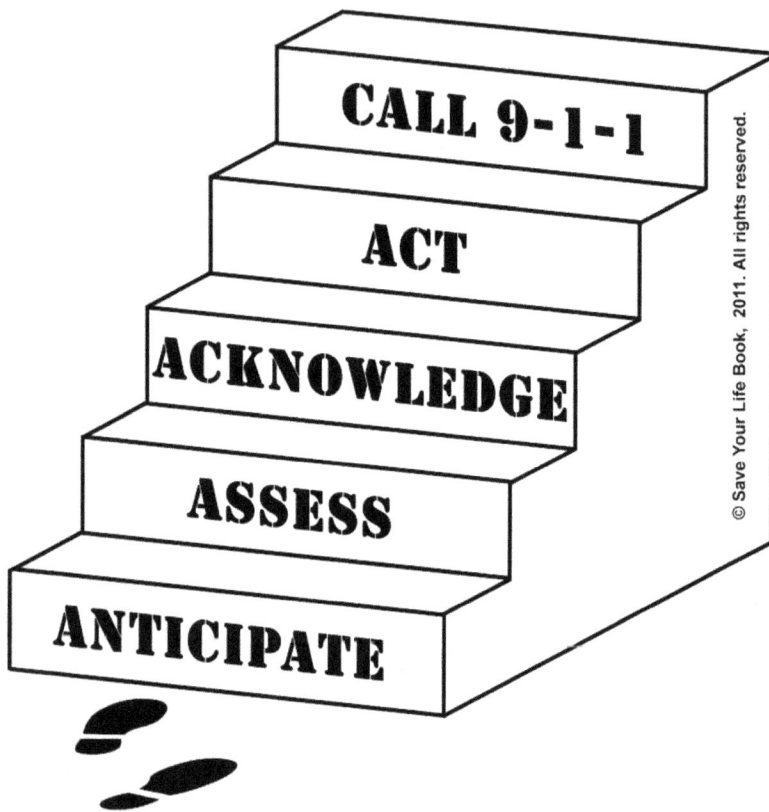

CALL 9-1-1

ACT

ACKNOWLEDGE

ASSESS

ANTICIPATE

ESSENTIAL STEPS TO ...

SAVE YOUR LIFE

www.ingramcontent.com/pod-product-compliance
Lightning Source LLC
Chambersburg PA
CBHW060029210326
41520CB00009B/1064